VOICES OF STRENGTH AND HOPE

Women's Stories of Overcoming Fibroids

Stories of Pain, Power, and
Healing from Fibroids

DR. QUANITA J. CRABLE, M.D.

Copyright © 2025 by Dr. Quanita Crable
All rights reserved. No part of this publication may be reproduced, distributed or transmitted in any form or by any means, including photocopying, recording or other electronic or mechanical means, without the proper written permission of the author or publisher, except in the case of brief quotations embodied in critical reviews and certain other noncommercial uses permitted by copyright law.

Disclaimer
The information provided in this eBook is intended for general knowledge and educational purposes only. It does not constitute medical advice. Please consult with a qualified healthcare professional for any health concerns or before making decisions related to your health or treatment.
The stories in this book reflect the author's recollection of events. Some names, minor details, and identifying characteristics have been changed to protect the privacy of those depicted.

Paperback ISBN: 979-8-9990115-0-3
Hardcover ISBN: 979-8-9990115-1-0

Published by

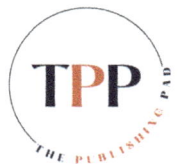

The Publishing Pad
www.thepublishingpad.com

What People Are Saying

"Reading this book felt like sitting with a group of brave women, hearing their struggles and triumphs. It's not just a medical book—it's a book on hope, resilience and the power of having a doctor who truly cares."
—**Tiffany S. Northern,** MHA, FACHE.
President of Texas Health Resources Frisco

"I highly recommend this book to any woman who has given up on her dreams of having children because of fibroids. I've been there. Dr. Crable's care gave me the confidence to believe in my body again, and this book will do the same for you."
—**Brit Rettig Wold**

"Dr. Crable beautifully captures the stories of real women from all seasons of life…. *Voices of Strength and Hope* is not only encouraging and hopeful but also informative."
—**Chloe**

"*Voices of Strength and Hope* is a culmination of the experience and wisdom the author has gained over the years. I hope women suffering from fibroids can find comfort and knowledge in her words."
—**Dr. Tiffanny Jones,** *M.D. Reproductive Endocrinologist*

"I highly recommend this book to any woman who has been diagnosed with fibroids, suspects she might have them, or to anyone who simply wants to be more informed about women's reproductive health."
—**LaDawna Crittenton McKinney,** *MHA, BSN, RNC-IAP, Best-selling Author*

"In *Voices of Strength and Hope,* Dr. Crable has seamlessly provided a voice for the often-dismissed faction of women who are often suffering in silence."
—**Maya Heath,** *M.D. Neonatologist*

Dedication

This book is for the women who came before me, the women beside me, and the women I fight for every day.

To my mother, Benita Duckett, my first home, my first teacher, my constant why. Without you, I wouldn't exist. But beyond giving me life, you gave me purpose. Watching your struggle lit a fire in me that's never gone out. Your pain became my calling. Your strength became my foundation. I carry your story in everything I do, and it's because of you that I will never stop fighting for women who deserve better.

To my grandmother, Dorester Montgomery, my best friend, my safe place, my greatest encourager. Your love was quiet but fierce, and your belief in me never wavered. Even when I doubted myself, you didn't. You kept me grounded in truth, held me up with prayer, and reminded me I was capable of doing hard things. I miss you more than words can say, but your spirit walks with me every step of this journey.

To the woman who has suffered in silence, who has cried herself to sleep, who has been dismissed, overlooked, or told to "just deal with it," this book is yours.

To the woman who's exhausted from the weight of unanswered questions, from bleeding that never ends, from pain that no one sees—this is for you.

To the woman who still dreams of becoming a mother, of reclaiming her health, of being heard and healed, this is for you, too. You are not alone. You never were.

And to God, thank You for choosing me, for trusting me, for using me. This work is not my own. Every skill I have, every life I touch, every woman I help, I do it through You. My favorite verse, Romans 8:28, reminds me that all things work together for the good of those who love the Lord and are called according to His purpose. I know I've been called. And I pray that everything in this book brings healing, hope, and a reminder that your story still matters.

Contents

What People Are Saying. iii

Acknowledgments ix

INTRODUCTION
The Promise
That Made Me. 1

Chapter 1
Unseen, Unspoken: Understanding Fibroids. 9

Chapter 2
Treatment Options
for Fibroids. 17

Chapter 3
Miracle in the Making. 23

Chapter 4
When Two
Battles Collide 27

Chapter 5
Light Beyond the Bleeding. 31

Chapter 6
Pain, Hope,
and Pregnancy 35

Chapter 7
Toxic Turns and Healing Paths 41

Chapter 8
The Diagnosis
No One Saw Coming. 47

Chapter 9
Precision and Preservation 51

Chapter 10
The Silent Growth, and the Loud Dream 57

Conclusion
Breaking the Silence, Together 63

Frequently Asked Questions (FAQ) 69

Resources 75

About the Author 77

Reviews 79

Acknowledgments

My deepest gratitude and appreciation to friends and first readers, Kellie Boyd, Felecia Green, and Latia Johnson, who shared their wisdom, insights, and time to help make this dream come true.

And thank you to my amazing team: Dr. Lisa Taylor-Kennedy (anesthesiologist), Lincy Mathew, Registered Nurse First-Assist, and Kathy Harrell, Certified Surgical Technologist. Without you all the journey would be harder.

INTRODUCTION
The Promise That Made Me

Ever since I could speak, I told anyone who would listen that I was going to be a doctor. I didn't just say it—I believed it, down to my core.

When I was a little girl, I would play doctor with my brother like it was the most natural thing in the world. My mother bought me a toy stethoscope, and I would walk with it around my neck, examining my brother like I had the power to heal. In my mind, I wasn't pretending—I was a doctor.

That dream only grew stronger with time, but it was forever cemented in my heart the day I lost my grandmother.

I was 16 when she died suddenly of a heart attack. She was only 59. One moment she was with us, and the next, she was gone. No warning. No goodbye.

The grief was unbearable. She was my heart. The one who always believed in me, always listened when I talked about being a doctor. I used to sit next to her, hold her hand, and say, "Grandma, I'm going to be a doctor one day." And she would smile and say, "I believe you, baby. I know you will."

When she passed, something shifted inside me. I felt like a part of me had been ripped away. But in that pain, I made a decision. I wasn't going to let her down. I was going to fulfill the promise I made to her. No matter how hard the road was, I was going to become a doctor—not just for me, but for her.

Growing up, I was always a bright student, though I had my moments. I wasn't a perfect child—I got in trouble sometimes, got sent to the principal's office, had a few stints in in-school suspension. But deep down, I knew I was capable of something greater. By the time I hit high school, I started to take things more seriously. My grades reflected that. I was excelling, especially in science and math. I was focused. Determined.

I remember one day, my counselor called me in and asked, "Quanita, do you plan to go to college?"

I smiled and said, "Yes, I'm going to be a doctor."

She nodded and handed me a paper. "Well, you need to take the SAT tomorrow. Tell your mom you need No. 2 pencils and a scientific calculator."

That was it—no prep, no guidance, no encouragement. Just a test the next morning that would help determine my future. But I showed up. I did what I had to do. And by God's grace, I scored well enough to earn a scholarship to the University of Kansas (KU).

Why KU? My brother went there, and that was good enough for me. I didn't know much about the school. I didn't do any research. I just knew that if my brother could do it, so could I. I followed in his footsteps, unknowingly walking into my purpose.

Getting to college was another last-minute scramble. My mother and I were trying to figure out forms, deadlines, financial aid—all the things no one had ever taught us. But we made it through.

Once I got to KU, I hit the ground running. I took advanced science and math courses and was a straight-A student. I felt good. I felt ready. When I scheduled my meeting with the pre-med advisor, I walked in with confidence.

But what happened next still sits with me.

He looked at me, didn't ask about my grades, didn't ask about my goals, and said, "I think medicine is going to be too hard for you. I don't think you're cut out for it. Let's look at some other career options."

I was stunned. Hurt. Confused. But most of all, I was angry. How could he say that? He didn't even know me.

I thought maybe it was a fluke, so I went to the second advisor he referred me to. But that meeting was no better. He echoed the same thing: "Let's find you another path."

In those moments, I realized I was going to have to fight, not just for my dream, but for the right to even pursue it.

Despite my grades, my commitment, and my passion, I was still being told I wasn't enough. But deep inside, I knew better. I'd already made a promise and I wasn't about to break it.

I took matters into my own hands. I started searching for opportunities, for guidance, for someone, anyone, who believed in me.

I had the opportunity to participate in a KU outreach program where we mentored inner-city kids in Kansas City, teaching them about science and math. That experience changed me. I saw myself in those kids. I saw how much potential they had and how much they needed someone to believe in them. Just like I did.

Through that program, I found the Health Career Pathways Program—a program for underserved and minority students who dreamed of becoming doctors. And when I say God knew what He was doing, I mean it. That program saved me.

It opened doors I never even knew existed. It gave me exposure to medicine, mentors who looked like me, and a community of students who understood the challenges I faced. It also offered me something priceless: the opportunity to interview for medical school at the University of Kansas—just for being in the program.

They helped me prepare for the MCAT. I studied hard. I did okay, not stellar, but solid.

What I didn't realize then was that I had severe test-taking anxiety. I wasn't alone—many brilliant people struggle with it. I knew the material. I was smart. But when it came time to test, panic would creep in. Even so, I did well enough to earn that interview.

I only got one interview. I only needed one.

And when I sat in that room with the admissions committee, I told them my truth. I told them about the little girl with the toy stethoscope. About my grandmother's death. About the promise I made, and the people who tried to steer me off course. I told them about my faith, my fight, and the fire in me that never burned out even when others tried to extinguish it.

I left that interview knowing I had spoken from my heart. Because sometimes, when the world says "no," your soul has to shout "yes" even louder.

After graduating from college, I moved back home and began working at a pharmacy. It wasn't my dream job, not by a long shot, but it was a stepping stone, a way to stay close to the world of medicine while I waited for the next door to open. I knew I wouldn't be there long. I had already set my heart on something far greater: medical school.

One day, I came home from work, and my mom met me with a familiar sparkle in her eye. "Quanita," she said, holding an envelope, "you got a letter from KU."

My heart stopped.

We sat together and opened it, hands trembling, breath held. I unfolded the letter, and in bold, beautiful words it read: "Congratulations, Quanita. You've been accepted to the University of Kansas School of Medicine."

I will never forget that moment. It was like time stood still. I screamed, cried, laughed—it all came pouring out. All the rejection, the doubt, the nights of silent prayer, the promise I made to my grandmother—it had all led to this moment. I knew then that God's plan for my life was not just real; it was unfolding.

I was so overwhelmed with joy that I couldn't contain it. I ran into work the next day beaming with pride and blurted out, "I got into medical school!"

My mother had warned me, "don't tell them yet, they'll let you go," but in my innocence and excitement, I couldn't keep it in.

She was right. The very next day, they fired me. But I didn't care. Because I was headed to medical school. I was stepping into my purpose.

When I began medical school, I was sure of one thing: I was going to be a cardiologist. After all, it was heart disease that took my grandmother from us far too soon. I was determined to save lives so that no one else would feel the pain I felt when she died.

But God had other plans.

During my second year of medical school, I faced a medical challenge of my own. I needed surgery—a gynecologic surgery to remove a cyst from my ovary. That was my first personal experience with the field of obstetrics and gynecology. It opened a door I hadn't considered before.

Around that same time, the women around me—friends and loved ones—were going through deeply personal battles. A close friend nearly lost her life to a GYN infection. Others were facing teen pregnancies. And my own mother, the woman who raised me with such strength, was suffering silently from fibroids—painful, debilitating, unrelenting fibroids that were taking over her body and her quality of life. Watching her suffer broke me in ways I can't describe. I felt helpless. But that helplessness quickly turned into motivation.

When I began my OB/GYN rotation during my third year, everything changed. I fell in love with the field. The variety. The urgency. The intimacy of caring for women through every stage of life. And more than anything, the power to help women like my mother—women living in pain, unheard and underserved.

Also around this time, I was finally diagnosed with test-taking anxiety—a silent struggle I didn't know had been following me for years. I wasn't struggling because I wasn't smart. I was struggling because fear gripped me in the moments I needed clarity the most. But with the help of a counselor and the courage to confront that fear, I learned how to manage it. From that moment forward, I aced every standardized exam I took.

I finished medical school, matched into an OB/GYN residency program, and—fittingly—I stayed right there at the University of Kansas, the very place where my journey began.

During my medical residency at the University of Kansas School of Medicine, I developed a strong interest in laparoscopic surgery—minimally invasive procedures that focus on the abdominal and pelvic organs. I found myself especially drawn to treating women with large fibroids. I saw how life-changing the relief could be.

I was trained by some of the most incredible surgeons in the country. Dr. Charles Alexander, may he rest in peace, taught me how to handle large fibroids; how to remove them with confidence, even if it meant opening the patient. He had this incredible way of trusting us to do the work, guiding us from the sidelines, shaping our hands and minds with his wisdom.

Then there was Dr. Madhuri Reddy, who taught me the art of laparoscopy—the grace and precision of minimally invasive surgery using the smallest incisions. She showed me how to bring healing with a gentler touch.

I took the strengths of both mentors and made them my own. I carried a laparoscopic box with me everywhere—practicing, sharpening, pushing myself to be better. I recorded every surgery and studied them obsessively. I watched my movements, studied my techniques, analyzed every choice I made in the operating room because I was determined to become great.

Then, in 2007, da Vinci robotic surgery was introduced to our program. I was immediately intrigued and worked tirelessly to become skilled in this cutting-edge technology. The da Vinci robotic system—named after Leonardo da Vinci, a pioneer of anatomical study—enables surgeons to perform highly precise, minimally invasive surgeries.

I studied. I practiced. I pushed myself. And eventually, I realized I could use this platform to treat even very large fibroids through small incisions. That discovery was a full-circle "aha" moment.

I had no idea then that I was destined to become a robotic fibroid surgeon. But once again, God was ahead of me.

And now, I remove fibroids the size of cantaloupes through incisions smaller than a dime. I use the robot as my tool of choice, a marvel of technology that allows me to offer hope to women who were once told they had no options.

Every patient I see reminds me why I do this. Some want to be mothers. Some just want the bleeding to stop. Some want their energy back. Their peace back. Their lives back.

If you're reading this book, it means you're dealing with fibroids or supporting someone who is. No matter what you need, I see you. I hear you. And I fight for you. Because I remember what it felt like to be unheard.

I remember the pain of losing someone I loved because no one saw the signs.

And I remember the promise I made to a 16-year-old girl with tears in her eyes and a dream in her heart.

That promise is why I'm here. That promise is why I have written this book.

This work is my calling. I walk in my purpose every day, using the skills I've been blessed with to offer women hope—real, tangible hope.

That's what this book is about—sharing the real stories of women who chose to reclaim their health, their hope, and their lives.

I'm honored to tell their stories.

And I'm humbled that God chose me as a vessel to help bring women back to wholeness. I hope that these stories will not only inspire you but also provide you with the tools to take back control of your life from the condition called fibroid.

Let's begin!

CHAPTER 1
Unseen, Unspoken: Understanding Fibroids

For far too long, fibroids have lived in the shadows of women's health—whispered about behind closed doors, brushed off as "just heavy periods," or dismissed entirely.

Millions of women suffer in silence, sometimes for years, not realizing that what they're going through is not normal. They bleed through clothes, miss work, avoid intimacy, carry pain in their backs, their pelvises, their bellies and often in their hearts.

My mother was a victim. She would often faint due to dangerously low blood levels caused by heavy bleeding. It was frightening to witness. Even after menopause stopped the bleeding, the cramping pain lingered. Watching her struggle for decades lit a fire in me—one that still burns today.

Fibroids are tumors that grow in or on the uterus. They're usuallynot cancerous, but for many women, they are life-altering.

They can cause heavy, prolonged bleeding, pelvic pressure, frequent urination, constipation, anemia, painful sex, infertility, and miscarriages. Some women develop such large fibroids that they appear several months pregnant. Others never know they have them until they're trying to get pregnant or until the symptoms become unbearable.

Studies show that up to 70-80% of women will develop fibroids by age 50. Of this number, 80% are black women and 70% are white women. Black women are disproportionately affected, often developing fibroids at younger ages, with larger, more numerous growths, and more severe symptoms.

Despite how common they are, fibroids are often misunderstood, misdiagnosed, or mismanaged. Far too many women are told that the only solution is a hysterectomy. Far too few are told about the full range of options available, including hormonal therapies, embolization, myomectomy, or advanced minimally invasive surgeries.

This chapter isn't about statistics, though. It's about visibility. It's about reclaiming the narrative around fibroids and giving voice to the women whose lives they've touched. This book is about the real stories—raw, honest, and hopeful—of women who found the strength to speak up, seek answers, and fight for their healing.

These stories matter because too often, fibroids steal more than just health. Fibroids steal confidence. Careers. Relationships. Dreams of motherhood. Peace of mind.

But they don't have to.

There are options. There is help. And most importantly, there is hope.

This chapter begins with knowledge, because knowledge is power. And the chapters that follow are filled with women who reclaimed that power—one voice, one surgery, one healing moment at a time.

Let their stories remind you: You are not alone. You are not invisible. And your pain is never "just part of being a woman."

The silent weight of fibroids

If fibroids had a sound, it would be the rustle of a woman changing pads every hour in a bathroom stall, afraid of leaking through her clothes again.

If they had a face, it would be the woman curled up on her couch, a heating pad pressed to her belly, canceling yet another plan with friends.

If they had a language, it would be silence—the kind passed down from mothers to daughters with warnings like, "We just have bad periods in this family."

Fibroids are far more than just growths in the uterus. They are more than bad periods. They are physical burdens, emotional drains, and often spiritual battles for the women who carry them.

What are fibroids?

Uterine fibroids, also known as leiomyomas or myomas, are non-cancerous tumors made of muscle and fibrous tissue.

They can range in size from tiny, undetectable nodules to massive growths that distort and enlarge the uterus. A woman can have one fibroid or dozens.

Fibroids grow in different parts of the uterus:

- **Intramural fibroids:** Develop within the muscular wall of the uterus.
- **Submucosal fibroids:** Grow just beneath the inner lining and can protrude into the uterine cavity, often causing the heaviest bleeding.
- **Subserosal fibroids:** Project to the outside of the uterus and can press on surrounding organs like the bladder or bowel.

- **Pedunculated fibroids:** Hang by a stalk either inside or outside the uterus.

Common symptoms of fibroids

Some women with fibroids have no symptoms at all. Others experience profound disruption in their lives. **Here are some of the most common symptoms reported by these women:**

- Heavy or prolonged menstrual bleeding
- Pelvic pressure or pain
- Frequent urination or urinary retention
- Constipation or bloating
- Pain during sex
- Anemia from blood loss
- Fatigue and low energy
- Difficulty getting pregnant or staying pregnant
- Enlarged abdomen (sometimes mistaken for weight gain or pregnancy)

Yet even with these life-altering symptoms, many women are misdiagnosed or not taken seriously. They are told to simply endure it as part of being a woman but this shouldn't be.

Why are fibroids so common and yet so mysterious?

Medical science doesn't fully understand what causes fibroids, but several risk factors are known:

- **Genetics:** Women with a family history of fibroids are more likely to develop them.
- **Hormones:** Estrogen and progesterone fuel fibroid growth. They often grow during reproductive years and shrink after menopause.
- **Race:** Black women are two to three times more likely to develop fibroids, often at younger ages and with more severe symptoms.
- **Health and Environment:** Obesity and diet may also play a role, along with vitamin D deficiency and environmental exposures.

Still, these are only pieces of a larger puzzle. Research into fibroids remains underfunded, and for too long, the condition has been under-discussed in medical education and public discourse alike.

Treatment options: one size does not fit all

You may have heard that hysterectomy is the only option for treating fibroids but that's simply not true. Thanks to advancements in technology, there are now several treatment options available, and the right one differs from person to person. The best option depends on many factors, including the size, number and location of the fibroids, as well as your symptoms, age, fertility goals, and overall health. Treatment should always be personalized and women should be fully informed about all the available options. Some options include:

- **Watchful waiting:** For women with small fibroids that aren't causing symptoms, immediate treatment may not be necessary.
- **Medications:** Hormonal therapies like GnRH agonists, birth control pills, or tranexamic acid can reduce bleeding or shrink fibroids temporarily.
- **Uterine fibroid embolization (UFE):** A radiologic procedure that blocks blood flow to the fibroids, causing them to shrink. While effective for some, it can carry risks, especially for women desiring future fertility.
- **Myomectomy:** Surgical removal of fibroids with preservation of the uterus. This can be done via hysteroscopy, laparoscopy, or robotic-assisted techniques like the da Vinci system.
- **Hysterectomy:** Complete removal of the uterus. This ends bleeding and eliminates fibroids permanently but is a life-altering decision that must be weighed carefully.

Yet many women are never told about all these options. Instead, they are rushed into decisions, often without time to ask questions, explore alternatives, or consider future goals like pregnancy.

This book was written to change that.

Because every woman deserves to understand what's happening inside her body. Every woman deserves the chance to choose healing that honors her values and her life. And every woman deserves to know: You are not alone.

Today, I provide comprehensive women's healthcare in Dallas, supporting women from adolescence through post-menopause. Nearly every day, I see women who are suffering from fibroids. Fortunately, I've been able to help thousands break free from the pain.

Some women are now able to get pregnant or carry a healthy pregnancy to term. Others find that their postmenopausal bleeding and pain vanish overnight. And for many, fibroid treatment brings an end to excruciating pain, constant bleeding, and the silent suffering of feeling misunderstood and dismissed. We will explore each of the options in the next chapter.

Myths about fibroids

Here are the most frequent myths about fibroids that I hear:

Myth: Fibroids always cause symptoms. Many women have fibroids without experiencing pain or heavy bleeding.

Myth: Hysterectomy is the only treatment option. There are multiple treatment approaches, including myomectomy and non-surgical methods.

Myth: Fibroids always cause infertility. Many women with fibroids conceive naturally or with treatment.

Myth: Fibroids shrink completely after menopause. Some fibroids persist and can still cause symptoms.

Myth: Fibroids turn into cancer. Fibroids are almost always benign, with a very low risk of malignancy.

Too often, women come to me feeling defeated, having been told:

- "You can't get pregnant."
- "You won't be able to carry a healthy pregnancy to term."
- "You have to have a hysterectomy."
- "You have to have open abdominal surgery."
- "Your fibroid removal might lead to complications that require an immediate hysterectomy."

But I tell them a different story. One of options. One of empowerment. One of healing.

With the right treatment, you can eliminate fibroids and the pain and discomfort they cause. We will look at all the options you have to be free from fibroids in the next chapter.

CHAPTER 2

Treatment Options for Fibroids

One of the most empowering aspects of living in today's world is the growing number of choices women have when it comes to managing their health. This is especially true for fibroids.

Not long ago, a hysterectomy was often the default recommendation. Today, there's a spectrum of treatment options, ranging from conservative management to advanced surgical techniques, that allow care to be personalized based on a woman's symptoms, reproductive goals, and preferences.

Fibroids don't affect every woman the same way, and because of that, there is no one-size-fits-all approach to treatment. Some women discover they have fibroids during a routine pelvic exam or imaging for another issue and they may never experience a single symptom. Others may live with debilitating pain, heavy bleeding, fatigue, infertility, or the emotional toll that comes from feeling unheard or misdiagnosed.

In this chapter, we will explore all the available treatment options. The right choice depends on your needs, but knowledge is power and knowing what's available is the first step toward reclaiming control over your body and your future.

1. **Watchful waiting (expectant management)**
   For women with small, asymptomatic fibroids, or those approaching menopause when fibroids tend to shrink naturally, watchful waiting may be the best option. No active treatment is done. Instead, regular monitoring with pelvic exams and ultrasounds ensures that any growth or development of symptoms is caught early.

   This path can be comforting for those who prefer a non-invasive approach, but it may not be the best option for women trying to conceive or those who've already experienced miscarriage or infertility. For them, a more proactive route may be necessary.

2. **Medications**
   Medications don't eliminate fibroids, but they can relieve symptoms like heavy bleeding, cramping, and anemia. Options include:

   - **Hormonal contraceptives (birth control pills, patches, vaginal rings):** They can help regulate periods and reduce bleeding.
   - **Hormonal Intrauterine Devices (IUDs) (like the levonorgestrel-releasing IUD):** IUDs are often used to reduce menstrual bleeding and cramping while providing birth control.
   - **Gonadotropin-releasing hormone (GnRH) agonists (e.g., leuprolide):** These drugs temporarily shrink fibroids by putting the body into a menopausal-like state. They can be useful before surgery to make fibroids easier to remove, or as a bridge to menopause in women nearing that phase.

- **Non-hormonal options:** Options such as tranexamic acid (Lysteda) or Nonsteroidal Anti-inflammatory Drugs (NSAIDs) can help manage bleeding and pain in select cases.

It's important to note that medications often provide temporary relief, and symptoms may return once treatment is stopped.

3. **Minimally invasive procedures**

   For women who want to avoid major surgery or preserve fertility, several minimally invasive options are available.

   - **Uterine Fibroid Embolization (UFE):** This radiologic procedure blocks the arteries feeding the fibroids, causing them to shrink. UFE is effective for symptom relief but can carry risks for future fertility and may not be ideal for women hoping to become pregnant.
   - **MRI-Guided Focused Ultrasound (MRgFUS):** This non-invasive technique uses high-intensity ultrasound waves to target and destroy fibroid tissue under MRI guidance. It has shown promise, especially for women who are not surgical candidates, though its availability may be limited and long-term outcomes are still being studied.
   - **Myomectomy:** This surgical procedure removes fibroids while preserving the uterus, making it ideal for women wanting to maintain fertility. Myomectomy can be performed in different ways:

     - **Laparoscopic or robotic-assisted myomectomy (minimally invasive):** Involves small incisions and faster recovery, but requires a highly skilled surgeon, especially for large or multiple fibroids.

- **Open abdominal myomectomy:** Involves a larger incision and longer recovery but is sometimes necessary for very large or numerous fibroids.
- **Hysteroscopic myomectomy:** Used for fibroids inside the uterine cavity, this approach involves no external incisions and offers a quick recovery.

Choosing the right type of myomectomy depends on the size, number, and location of the fibroids, as well as the surgeon's expertise.

4. **Hysterectomy**

   Hysterectomy, or the surgical removal of the uterus, is the only treatment that guarantees fibroids will not return. While it may be the best option for some, especially those with severe symptoms or other uterine conditions, it is a major decision with lifelong implications. There are several types:

- Total hysterectomy (removal of the uterus and cervix)
- Subtotal (supracervical) hysterectomy (removal of the uterus while leaving the cervix intact)
- Hysterectomy with bilateral salpingectomy or oophorectomy (removal of fallopian tubes and/or ovaries if needed)

Minimally invasive approaches, including robotic-assisted and laparoscopic hysterectomy, have greatly improved recovery times and outcomes, making this procedure safer and less traumatic than in the past.

However, this option is typically reserved for women who are done with childbearing or whose fibroids are causing extreme symptoms that haven't responded to other treatments.

Emerging and future treatments

Innovation in fibroid treatment continues to evolve, offering hope for more effective, less invasive solutions:

1. **Radiofrequency ablation (RFA)**
   This procedure destroys fibroid tissue using controlled heat. It can be done laparoscopically or via a device called Sonata. Early results are promising, especially for symptom relief and faster recovery.

2. **Selective progesterone receptor modulators (SPRMs)**
   These drugs target hormone receptors on fibroid cells, potentially shrinking fibroids while controlling bleeding.

3. **Stem cell and gene-based research**
   Scientists are beginning to understand the genetic and cellular roots of fibroids, potentially paving the way for curative treatments in the future.

Choosing the right treatment: you have a voice

Every woman's fibroid journey is unique. You may need to try different treatments, get a second opinion, or take time to process your options before making a decision. It's okay to ask questions, seek out specialists, or advocate for a less invasive or uterus-preserving path if that's what you desire.

Your body. Your choice. Your journey.

In the chapters that follow, you'll read the stories of women, just like you, who explored different treatment options and found healing from fibroids. They are now living healthier, fuller lives. My hope is that one day, I'll get to share your story too.

CHAPTER 3

Miracle in the Making

Ashley Burnett was only 20 years old when she first encountered the sharp, breath-stealing pain that would forever change her life. She was rushed to the emergency room, doubled over and terrified.

"I was experiencing pain, crippling pain, to where I had to go into the emergency room," she later shared in an interview with CBS News Texas. "That's when I discovered that I had fibroids."

At 20, Ashley was too young to be thinking about reproductive health challenges. She had dreams, plans for her future, and a vision of motherhood that felt far away but certain. But the diagnosis shook that certainty. What began as a medical discovery would evolve into a 15-year battle with fibroids—tumors that would test her strength, patience, and faith.

When Ashley walked into my office, it had been years since that first ER visit. She was now in her mid-30s, married, and aching from a recent pregnancy loss.

At 22 weeks' gestation, just past the halfway mark, she had lost a baby she had already begun to love with her whole heart.

The devastation of that loss was magnified by the knowledge that the fibroids she had fought to control—those same fibroids that had caused her years of pain—might have been the reason her baby didn't survive.

Ashley had undergone a procedure prior to her pregnancy to shrink the fibroids. She had done everything right. She had followed the recommendations, listened to doctors, and still, the loss came.

When she sat across from me in my office, she was scared, emotionally raw, and clinging to hope by a thread.

Her periods weren't unusually heavy, but the fibroids had grown silently and steadily, intruding on the space that should have been a safe haven for her baby.

"It's hard to share space," I told her gently. "Unfortunately, it's difficult for fibroids and a baby to coexist."

Fibroids can distort the uterine cavity, affect blood flow, and reduce the chances of a pregnancy making it to full term. In many women, they are a hidden cause of infertility or miscarriage, conditions often brushed off or misdiagnosed.

Ashley and I talked for a long time. She needed answers. She needed a plan. Most of all, she needed someone to believe that motherhood was still within reach.

We discussed her options in detail, with a focus on a minimally invasive robotic myomectomy.

The goal: remove the fibroids while preserving her uterus and giving her the best chance at a healthy pregnancy in the future. She understood the risks. She knew that a Cesarean delivery would be required in any future pregnancy, and that fibroids could return. But in that moment, hope outweighed fear.

Ashley underwent surgery, and I removed 26 fibroids from her uterus—twenty-six growths that had stolen years from her life and nearly taken her dream of becoming a mother.

One of her fallopian tubes was damaged and had to be removed. It was a complex surgery, but thanks to robotic technology and a minimally invasive approach, her recovery was smooth, and the integrity of her uterus was preserved.

Seven months later, Ashley returned to my office—this time with tears of joy. She was pregnant again.

That pregnancy went full term. And so did the next.

Today, Ashley is a mother of two: a beautiful daughter and a vibrant, healthy son. Her home is filled with the laughter of children and the soft, grateful rhythm of a dream realized. She and her husband are raising their family with love, deep appreciation, and with the memory of what they overcame to get here.

Going beyond medicine

Ashley's story is not just about medicine. It's about perseverance. It's about the power of second opinions, of not settling for unanswered questions, of advocating for yourself in a system that too often dismisses women's pain.

"There are so many women out there with my story," Ashley said. "And I just want this to be in the forefront, because I don't think people really realize how many women suffer with this… or lose a baby because of this."

Her story is a rallying cry. It's a reminder that fibroids aren't just a "women's health issue"—they are a public health issue, a family issue, a deeply human issue.

"Twenty-six fibroids later and one fallopian tube gone," Ashley says with quiet pride, "I still conceived. So don't give up."

CHAPTER 4

When Two Battles Collide

Kellie Boyd is more than my nurse and office manager—she is my best friend.

She has stood beside me during countless patient visits, long surgeries, and late-night phone calls. But behind her calm presence and professional strength was a quiet storm she had endured for years, an invisible, relentless battle with both fibroids and endometriosis.

I watched her suffer in silence, wearing a brave face while enduring a war inside her body.

Endometriosis, when the tissue similar to the lining of the uterus grows outside of it, can be debilitating. It affects about 10 to 15% of women of reproductive age, and up to 50% of women facing infertility. When combined with fibroids, the effects can be devastating. A study by the National Institutes of Health revealed that about 20% of women with symptomatic fibroids also have endometriosis. Kellie was one of them.

Each month, her period brought on a familiar agony. The bleeding was so heavy that she required a super-plus tampon along with two overnight pads, every single hour, for the first three to four days of her seven-day cycle. Her bathroom breaks were more about survival than routine.

There were countless moments when she bled through her clothes, moments filled with shame and frustration. And those moments were happening every 21 days.

The pain wasn't just physical—it consumed Kellie. It was the kind of pain that made her vomit, curl into a ball on the floor, and miss out on life. It stripped Kellie of energy, drained her joy, and left her managing her shifts through sheer willpower and a cocktail of ibuprofen. She took more painkillers in one week than I took in an entire year.

She tried everything—heating pads, yoga, elimination diets, supplements, lifestyle changes.

Nothing worked.

Nothing touched the deep, searing ache that radiated through her pelvis and settled in her bones. And while these efforts showed her commitment to healing, they only provided temporary, shallow relief.

At one point, Kellie radically shifted her diet. She cut out sugar, caffeine, dairy, and meat. She hoped each change would bring healing. And while there was a slight improvement, it was never enough. The bleeding still came, the pain still stabbed, and the exhaustion remained.

But Kellie is a nurse. She knew the limitations of what she was facing. And she knew there was something more powerful available—something that could actually give her life back.

In 2014, she made the courageous decision to undergo surgery, robotic-assisted surgery, to treat both her fibroids and her stage 4 endometriosis. She knew the risks. She also knew the rewards. Her body had cried out for too long, and it was time to answer.

During her surgery, multiple fibroids were removed, and widespread endometriosis was excised . What many don't realize is how often these two conditions coexist. In about 70 to 80% of cases, when we go in to remove fibroids, we find endometriosis lurking, too. And when we find it, we treat it.

Kellie enjoyed several years of peace following her first surgery. Her periods normalized, her pain subsided, and for the first time in years, she felt free. But fibroids and endometriosis are persistent. They do not always stay away.

In 2024, the symptoms crept back. The bleeding returned. The pain knocked again. But this time, Kellie didn't hesitate. She became the second person in the country to undergo surgery using the advanced da Vinci 5 surgical system.

We performed a second robotic myomectomy and resected her endometriosis once again. The procedure went smoothly. Her recovery was swift. She maintained her diet, stayed committed to her supplements, and most importantly, held on to the hope that she deserved a pain-free life.

That flicker of hope

Kellie once told me something that still echoes in my mind:

"Endometriosis and fibroids stole so many of my moments—hope hijacked, joy interrupted, pain and bleeding that came like a thief in the night. There were days I spoke up, and days I said nothing at all. The pain made me angry, irritable, withdrawn. Sometimes I was loud. Sometimes I was quiet. But never was I looking for pity. I was trying to survive something no one else could see."

It was raw. It was real. It was the truth so many women live with.

But Kellie never gave up. Not on her body. Not on her healing. Not on her hope.

"And still, I held on to the flicker," she said. "That quiet flicker of hope that healing was possible. If you search for the right provider, advocate for yourself, and believe that your body still deserves peace, you will find the light again. And this time, it will shine brighter than the pain ever did."

Kellie's story is a testament to the resilience of women everywhere who fight battles no one sees. It's a reminder that our pain is real, that our voices matter, and that healing is not only possible, it's worth fighting for.

I am incredibly proud of Kellie. She continues to show up for herself, and for so many others, every single day.

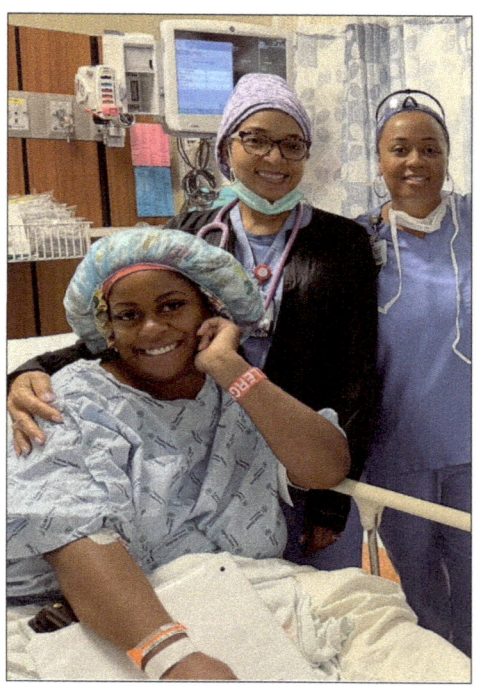

CHAPTER 5

Light Beyond the Bleeding

Felecia Green was no stranger to hospitals. As a seasoned nurse, she had comforted patients, held hands through difficult diagnoses, and advocated fiercely for others. But when her own health began to unravel, she found herself in unfamiliar territory—on the other side of the conversation, seeking answers that no one seemed to have.

I first met Felecia in the corridors of the hospital where we both worked. She carried herself with a calm authority, always composed, always compassionate. So, when she pulled me aside one day, her voice lower than usual, I knew something was weighing heavily on her.

"I think I need your help," she said quietly. "The bleeding… it hasn't stopped."

Felecia was in her mid-50s, well past menopause. She had expected this new stage of life to bring relief—no more monthly cycles, no more cramping, and no more inconvenience. Instead, she found herself trapped in a cycle of confusion and fear.

"Postmenopausal bleeding. I never thought those words would apply to me," Felecia told me later. "Menopause had come and gone. I should've been free of all that. But then one day, there was spotting. A few weeks later, light bleeding. It came and went, sometimes with cramping, always with dread."

She did the responsible thing. She saw her doctor, someone she had trusted for three decades, who performed a biopsy.

Thankfully, the results were normal. But her uterine lining was thickened, a finding that raised quiet concern in her mind.

Her doctor reassured her: "Let's just watch and wait."

So, she waited. And the bleeding didn't stop.

"Every time I saw blood, I panicked," Felecia said. "What if it's cancer? What if we're waiting too long? What if I'm not being taken seriously?"

Felecia's instincts, sharpened by years working in healthcare, told her something was not right. Despite the reassurance from her doctor and the normal biopsy, her symptoms persisted and so did her anxiety.

"I was tired of feeling like I had to convince someone that I knew my body," she said. "And I realized—I didn't have to stay in that place."

Though her gynecologist had been managing her with birth control pills and performing frequent, painful biopsies, one key diagnostic step had never been taken: no one had ordered a pelvic sonogram.

That's when Felecia heard about me from a colleague, a friend, a patient who shared her fibroid story.

"They said Dr. Crable listens," Felecia recalled. "And that's what I needed more than anything.

"People spoke about her kindness, her skill, and most importantly, her willingness to listen, so I made an appointment. From the moment I met her, I felt something different—she truly heard me. She didn't dismiss my concerns. Instead, she gave me simple but powerful advice: 'Let's start with a sonogram.' That one step changed everything. The scan revealed multiple fibroids, including one pressing against my bladder, likely causing both the abnormal bleeding and my frequent urination. It was more than I had ever been told before. It was the answer I had been waiting for."

Felecia's sonogram showed large uterine fibroids that she had no idea existed. She was tired of bleeding, painful biopsies, and taking birth control pills on a repeat cycle, so she decided to have a minimally invasive robotic hysterectomy.

After a hysterectomy performed this way, the most important restrictions are no lifting over 10 to 15 pounds, and nothing in the vagina (tampons, douches, or intercourse) for six to eight weeks.

To this day, Felecia states that this surgery is one of the best decisions she has ever made.

"After 30 years with the same physician, I transferred my care to Dr. Crable, because for the first time, I felt like my health truly mattered," Felecia said. "The procedure was smooth, my recovery was quick, and within two weeks, I was back to work. More than the surgery itself, what changed my life was knowing that someone cared enough to listen, to act, and to make sure I received the care I truly needed."

CHAPTER 6

Pain, Hope, and Pregnancy

Pregnancy is often described as a time of glowing anticipation and tender milestones.

For Shante Jackson, however, her first pregnancy became a season of heartbreak wrapped in physical pain. Her experience was anything but typical. It was shaped by the silent burden of uterine fibroids that were large enough to threaten both her health and her baby's chance at life.

Shante came to our office during her first pregnancy, full of hope and optimism. She had made it through the first trimester without incident, and she was just starting to show.

But a routine scan revealed a harsh reality: her uterus was home not only to her growing baby, but also to several very large fibroids—benign tumors that had quietly taken up residence and were now threatening to overshadow her pregnancy.

In her second trimester, Shante began experiencing intense pelvic pressure and intermittent pain, far more than the usual discomforts of pregnancy.

At just 15 weeks, we discovered her cervix had already started to shorten. The diagnosis was cervical insufficiency, a condition where the cervix opens too soon under the weight of a growing pregnancy. We acted quickly, placing a vaginal cerclage, a suture meant to reinforce the cervix and prevent premature birth.

Even with the cerclage in place, Shante's fibroids continued to grow, stretching her uterus and crowding the small space where her baby was supposed to thrive. The environment became hostile.

Within a week of her procedure, Shante lost her pregnancy. Her pain shifted from physical to emotional—the grief of losing her child so unexpectedly was devastating.

Despite all of this, however, Shante was determined not to give up. After mourning her loss and taking time to heal, she returned, resolute in her desire to one day carry a pregnancy to term.

This time, we created a proactive plan.

Shante underwent a robotic-assisted myomectomy—a minimally invasive surgery that allowed us to remove the large fibroids while preserving the integrity of her uterus. The precision of robotic surgery meant less bleeding, faster recovery, and most importantly, a better chance for Shante to conceive again.

And we didn't stop there.

Given Shante's history of cervical insufficiency, we also performed an abdominal cerclage, a more permanent and higher-strength suture placed during the robotic-assisted surgery. While vaginal cerclage has modest success rates, abdominal cerclage has been shown to prevent preterm birth in more than 90% of patients. In my own practice, I'm proud to say that number is even higher: 100%.

Shante embraced the plan with courage, and after a six-month recovery, she conceived again.

This time, Shante's pregnancy unfolded like a different story. With the fibroids gone and her cervix reinforced, Shante was finally able to experience the quiet joy of feeling her baby grow without fear of premature labor.

At 24 weeks, we gave her betamethasone, a steroid injection to accelerate the baby's lung development, just in case. Her care was meticulous and highly personalized every step of the way.

At 37 weeks, Shante gave birth via a planned Cesarean section, a precautionary decision to protect her uterus from rupture after prior surgeries. The birth was smooth, and the moment Shante heard her baby cry for the first time was a moment of redemption—a dream deferred, now finally realized.

Today, Shante is the proud mother of not just one, but three beautiful, healthy children.

Years later, Shante found herself facing a new challenge.

The fibroids had returned. While they were not as large as before, they were still disruptive. Shante began experiencing heavy bleeding, fatigue, and a deep, dull ache that lingered in her pelvis.

Shante had fulfilled her dream of building a family.

Now, she was ready for a different kind of freedom—freedom from pain, constant bleeding, and the looming worry of recurring fibroids.

After thoughtful consideration, Shante decided to have a robotic-assisted total laparoscopic hysterectomy, once again choosing the least invasive, most precise path forward. She also elected for a bilateral salpingectomy, which is the removal of both fallopian tubes, a decision that lowered her risk for ovarian cancer while preserving her hormone-producing ovaries.

Shante recovered beautifully, and more importantly, she was finally able to live without the burden of fibroids, without pain or fear.

A voice for individualized care

Today, Shante is thriving. Her journey, filled with heartbreak, resilience, and ultimately, triumph, is a testament to the power of personalized medicine. No two women experience fibroids in the same way, and no two treatment paths are identical.

Shante's story reminds us that women deserve care tailored to their needs, their goals, and their dreams. And with today's technology, expertise, and empathy, that level of care is more accessible than ever.

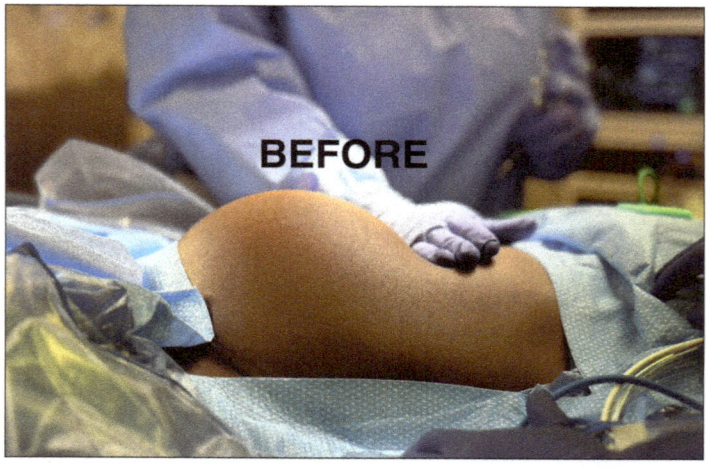

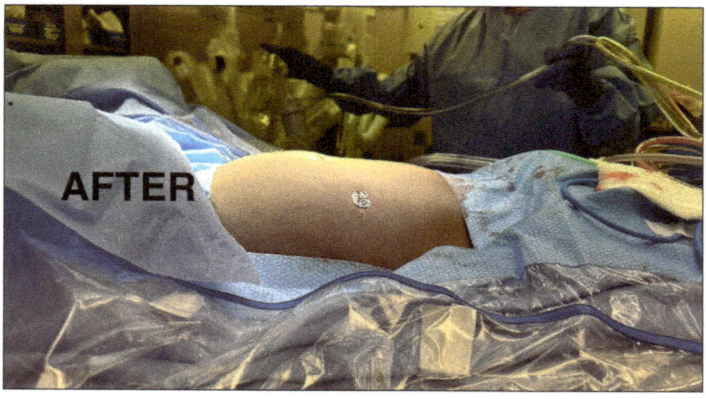

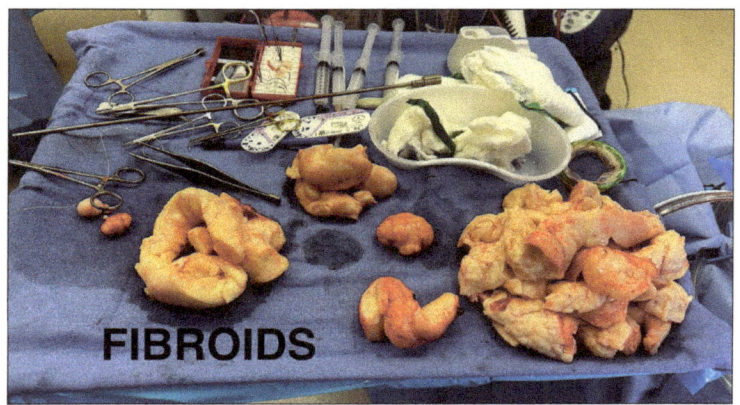
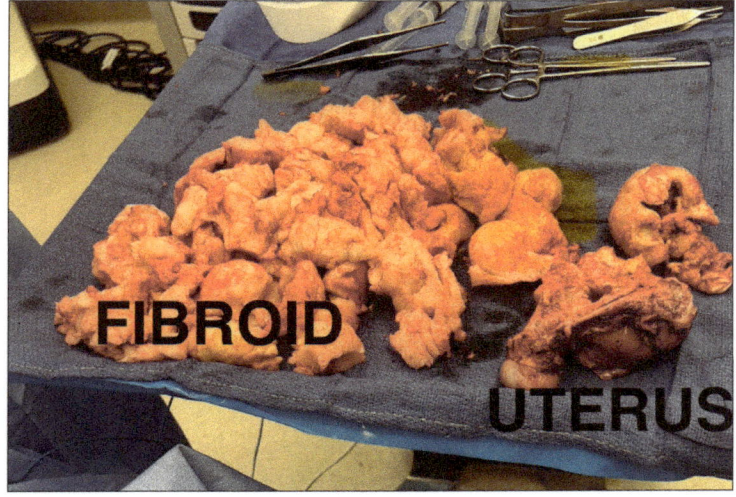
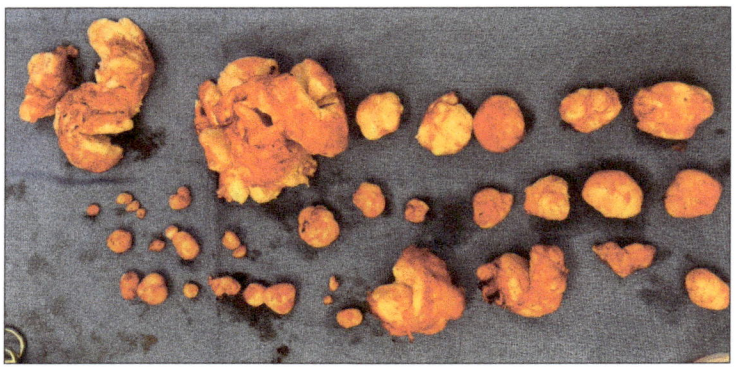

CHAPTER 7

Toxic Turns and Healing Paths

Not every woman's journey with fibroids begins in a gynecologist's office. For many, like Carla Franklin, the road to answers is long, winding, and filled with detours through other medical specialties.

Abdominal pain. Lower back aches. Heavy, soul-sapping bleeding. These symptoms often get sliced into separate diagnoses—digestive issues, sciatica, hormonal changes—before anyone stops to look at the uterus.

Carla was referred to me by an interventional radiologist when she was in her late 40s, worn down by years of pain, discomfort, and uncertainty. She had tried so many things, but still she suffered. She was a vibrant woman who loved to laugh. She showed up to our first appointment wearing a colorful scarf and bright lipstick, but beneath that cheerful armor was someone who had been living in the shadows of her own body.

Carla's fibroids weren't just a nuisance; they were a force that had completely altered her life. Her uterus had nearly grown to the size of a full-term pregnancy, pressing against her bladder and bowels, distorting her shape, and stealing her energy. Imagine walking around every day with the weight and pressure of a baby inside you, but without the joy of new life to balance the burden.

She had already undergone a procedure called Uterine Fibroid Embolization (UFE), a non-surgical option meant to shrink fibroids by cutting off their blood supply. For some women, UFE offers relief. But for Carla, it didn't. Her fibroids didn't shrink enough. The pain didn't go away. The bleeding didn't stop. Her abdomen still bulged out, drawing the wrong kind of stares and comments from strangers who assumed she was pregnant. It was humiliating, isolating, and confusing.

When I first met Carla, I remember how calmly she explained her history, much like someone who had rehearsed her story far too many times. She smiled politely, but the weariness in her voice betrayed how deeply this journey had drained her. We talked openly about her options, and she decided to move forward with a robotic-assisted laparoscopic hysterectomy and bilateral salpingectomy. We would preserve her ovaries, since she hadn't yet gone through menopause.

She was relieved to have a plan finally.

I showed her photos of other women who had undergone similar procedures, their before-and-after transformations, not just physically but emotionally. She teared up as she looked at them. "They look free," she whispered. "That's all I want—to feel free again."

We scheduled her surgery for a few months later, and she left my office hopeful for the first time in years.

But life had other plans.

A month later, my office phone rang. It was Carla. Her voice trembled. "I'm not okay," she said. "Something is really wrong." She had developed intense pain, fevers, chills, and a foul-smelling vaginal discharge that she described, with a painful laugh, as "so bad it's stinking up the entire house."

She had gone to the ER multiple times. Each time, she was told there was no sign of infection, and she was sent home. But Carla knew her body. She knew something was very, very wrong. And this time, she didn't let anyone dismiss her.

"Please," she said, "I feel like I'm dying."

I brought her into the office immediately. The moment she walked in, I knew we were in emergency territory. Her skin was pale, her eyes dull with exhaustion, her body clearly in distress. I admitted her straight to the hospital.

Tests confirmed what Carla already suspected in her gut: she was septic. Her fibroids had become infected, turning her uterus into a ticking time bomb. Her body was waging a war against itself, trying desperately to contain an infection that had already begun to spread.

She was started on IV antibiotics that same hour, and we fast-tracked her surgery.

Three days later, Carla was wheeled into the operating room for an emergency robotic total laparoscopic hysterectomy with bilateral salpingectomy. The surgery was difficult. Her uterus was massive, inflamed, and infected. Every move required precision. But we were prepared, and our team was ready.

I remember the moment we removed her uterus, sealed within a surgical bag and extracted through her belly button. It was surreal. That organ had stolen years of her life, distorted her body and her spirit and now, it was gone.

Carla stayed in the hospital for three more days under close supervision as her body healed. The change was almost immediate. The fevers stopped. Her white blood cell counts normalized. The pain, both physical and emotional, began to lift.

When I visited her post-op, she was sitting upright, eating Jell-O and chatting with the nurse. Her mother was by her side, tears in her eyes, holding Carla's hand like she never wanted to let go.

"I feel lighter," Carla told me, her voice cracking again. "Not just in my body… but everywhere. I feel like I'm finally waking up."

A new beginning

Carla's recovery continued to be smooth, thanks to the minimally invasive approach. Her scars were small, her pain manageable, and her spirits high.

But more than anything, Carla's story became a reminder, for me, and everyone around her, of the importance of listening to women. Of taking their symptoms seriously. Of trusting them when they say, "This isn't normal."

Embolization failure isn't often talked about (this occurs when the fibroids don't shrink as expected or symptoms return after a uterine fibroid embolization procedure). With its risks and delayed complications, it is not the happy, non-surgical fix many hope it will be. For Carla, it became something far worse.

But in the end, her strength won. Her voice saved her life. Her refusal to give up even when doctors told her she was fine carried her through the darkest part of her journey.

Carla's story is not just one of survival. It's one of reclaiming: reclaiming her body, her dignity, and her future. And through it all, she reminds us that even when fibroids try to steal everything, healing is still possible.

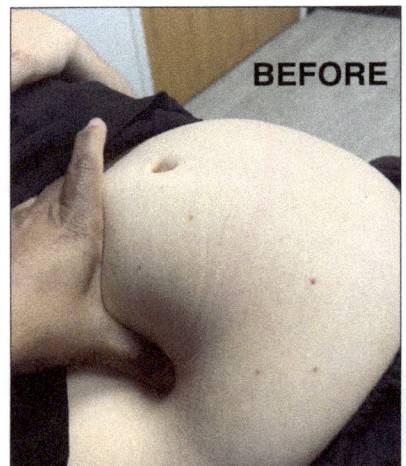
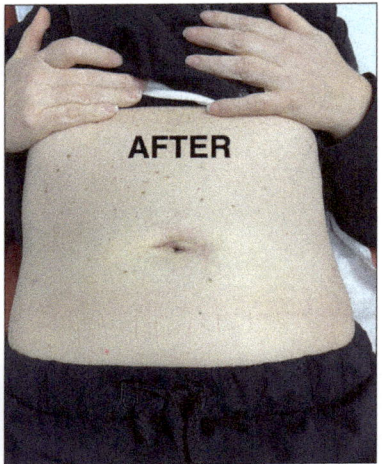
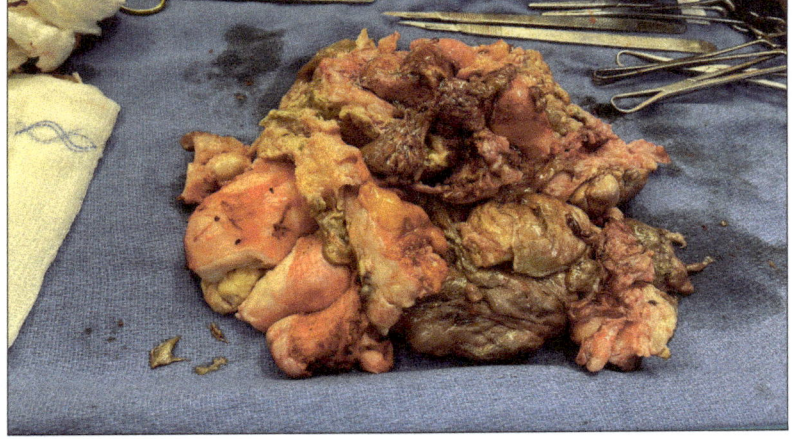

CHAPTER 8

The Diagnosis No One Saw Coming

Sondra Rose first came to me not just as a new patient, but as someone who already had a connection to my care—I had delivered her granddaughter.

I still remember the joy in her daughter's eyes as she cradled her baby for the first time. That shared moment of new beginnings became the foundation of the trust Sondra would later place in me when it came time to face something far more uncertain.

But when she first walked into my office, there was something quiet and heavy in her presence, an unspoken worry she'd carried for too long.

"I wasn't going to come," she told me later. "I thought maybe it would go away, or that I was overreacting. But deep down, I knew something wasn't right."

Sondra had been experiencing postmenopausal bleeding, an unnerving symptom that no woman should ignore. After a full year without a menstrual cycle, any bleeding becomes a red flag. It may be light, even barely noticeable, but its presence speaks loudly. For doctors, the concern is immediate: Could this be endometrial cancer?

It had taken Sondra months to gather the courage to make that call. So many women hesitate, not because they don't care about their health, but because of fear. Fear of hearing bad news. Fear of losing their sense of identity. Fear of surgery. She was no different. But she was brave enough to come.

At that first appointment, I completed a thorough evaluation. Sondra's imaging told a startling story: her uterus had grown to the size of a 33-week pregnancy—massive, especially for someone postmenopausal.

We performed an endometrial biopsy, a procedure that can be emotionally triggering for many women, especially when done in-office. Sondra gripped the exam table tightly, breathing through the discomfort. "I just kept praying it wouldn't be cancer," she later shared.

Thankfully, her biopsy came back benign; there was no cancer in the uterine lining. But the size of the fibroids, combined with her postmenopausal status, made the decision clear: Her uterus had to come out. I ordered an MRI to rule out any signs of advanced disease, but nothing overtly suspicious appeared.

We talked about the options: open surgery, laparoscopic, and the robotic-assisted approach. Sondra was relieved when I explained we could do the procedure with a minimally invasive approach using the robot. But I didn't sugarcoat the risks. We talked openly about the rare, but real, possibility of a hidden cancer.

"I didn't want to hear that word, cancer, but I appreciated that you didn't hide it from me. I needed the truth," she said.

Sondra went into surgery with grace and quiet strength. Despite her uterus weighing nearly six pounds, an enormous mass for a minimally invasive operation, we completed her hysterectomy robotically, with precision and care.

To protect her from the risk of tissue spreading, we used a containment bag, removing the uterus intact. We also removed both ovaries and fallopian tubes, reducing future cancer risk even further.

The surgery was long but uneventful, and Sondra woke up tired but relieved. She only stayed in the hospital for one night. Her incisions were tiny, no bigger than the width of the tip of my first finger.

At her first postoperative visit, Sondra was radiant: She was healing beautifully, moving with more ease, and smiling for the first time in weeks.

"I didn't realize how much pressure I had been living with," she said. "It was like my body had been trying to tell me something for years."

A week later, I received her final pathology report and my heart sank.

Buried within the fibroid-laden tissue was something none of us expected: a leiomyosarcoma. This is an aggressive, rare cancer that arises from the smooth muscle of the uterus. It affects fewer than 1% of women with fibroids, and it's nearly impossible to detect before surgery.

The weight of those words, leiomyosarcoma, carried so much fear and urgency. I called Sondra immediately.

She came into my office the next day, calm but searching my face for answers. I sat down with her and explained the results as gently and clearly as I could.

"I was shocked. I thought the worst was over. But then you told me… cancer," she recalled. "I remember feeling numb. Then I felt grateful because we had already taken it out."

Her imaging was clear. No signs of spread. The surgery, done with careful containment and precision, had likely saved her life.

To be certain, I referred Sondra to a gynecologic oncologist. I made the calls myself, ensuring the handoff was smooth. She started chemotherapy shortly afterward, not because there were signs of recurrence, but to be safe.

Chemotherapy is no small feat. It tests a woman's spirit. But Sondra handled it with the same grace she'd carried all along.

"I lost my hair. I lost some weight. But I never lost my faith," she told me during a follow-up.

And she never lost her spark.

Five years later: thriving and cancer-free

Today, Sondra is five years out, cancer-free, full of life, and stronger than ever. At every annual visit, she walks in with a confident stride and a warm hug.

She is a living testament to what can happen when women advocate for themselves, when they choose to face the unknown. When care is approached with compassion, precision, and partnership.

Sondra's story is rare. But it reminds us of a powerful truth: Even something as common as fibroids can carry hidden dangers. And while most fibroids are benign, women deserve thorough care. They deserve choices. They deserve honesty.

"I tell everyone now—don't wait. Don't ignore your body. You're worth the care," she says.

Her journey is one of courage. Of listening to the quiet alarm in her body. Of trusting her instincts. And of never giving up on the future.

CHAPTER 9

Precision and Preservation

Sometimes, women need to listen to their bodies and intuition and seek a second opinion. Sometimes, they need to get a third opinion, and in Jamie Scott's case, it was a fourth opinion that made all the difference.

There's something powerful, almost sacred, about a woman listening to her body. That quiet knowing, the whisper that something isn't right, the refusal to be dismissed. For Jamie, that inner voice wouldn't quiet down. And thank God it didn't.

Jamie was in her early 40s when she first walked into my office. From the outside, she looked composed, polished, and strong but just beneath the surface, she was carrying years of pain, frustration, and uncertainty.

Heavy menstrual bleeding tormented her every month. Pelvic pain left her curled up in bed with a heating pad more often than she cared to admit. The cramping was so intense that it felt like her uterus was trying to tear itself apart.

Jamie had to plan her life around bathroom breaks because her bladder never felt empty, and constipation made even simple meals feel like a gamble.

These weren't occasional nuisances. They were daily obstacles, slowly eroding her quality of life. And deep down, Jamie knew what was wrong. She suspected fibroids, just like her mother and aunt had faced. But what she didn't expect was the resistance she would face in getting the care she truly needed.

She had already seen three different OB/GYNs before she came to me. Each time, she walked into those offices hoping for understanding, maybe even a solution that matched her hopes. But all she received were the same tired words: "You need a hysterectomy." No conversation. No consideration. No alternatives.

Jamie hadn't had children yet. And though time wasn't on her side, she wasn't ready to close that chapter, not without a fight.

"I kept thinking… how can they just take away my uterus like it's nothing?" she told me, her voice trembling. "Like my dreams don't matter. Like I don't matter."

That's when she found me. Her fourth opinion. Her final hope.

We sat down together, and for the first time in this journey, Jamie felt heard. She wasn't rushed. She wasn't dismissed. Just heard.

Her imaging confirmed what she feared: multiple large fibroids, including one that was deeply embedded in her lower uterine segment, extending into the cervix. This wasn't just any fibroid. It was massive, over 10 centimeters, and wedged in a location that made surgical removal not only difficult but risky.

But Jamie wasn't scared, she was determined. "If there's a way to keep my uterus, I want to try," she said.

We talked at length about the procedure. I explained the challenges—how the cervical fibroid might impact the uterus-cervix connection, the potential for bleeding, and the importance of precision.

She asked thoughtful, sometimes heartbreaking questions. Could she still have children? What if it didn't work? What if this was her last chance?

With eyes full of hope and a heart full of courage, Jamie gave her consent. We scheduled a robotic myomectomy.

Surgery day arrived, and as I entered the operating room, I carried Jamie's hope with me. This wasn't just another case. It was a woman's future resting in our hands.

As expected, the large cervical fibroid dominated the lower uterus. It was like trying to extract a boulder from a narrow cave. During the delicate dissection, the right side of Jamie's uterus separated from her cervix. It was a heart-stopping moment. Any misstep could jeopardize her fertility, or worse.

But robotic surgery offers unmatched precision, and years of experience guided my hands. I gently realigned the tissue, meticulously reattaching the uterus to the cervix.

To support healing and reduce the risk of internal scarring, I placed a Foley catheter into the uterus—a move we hadn't discussed pre-op, but one I knew was necessary. A Foley catheter is a thin, flexible tube used to drain urine and monitor urine output.

One by one, I removed the other fibroids, each close to 10 centimeters. By the end of surgery, Jamie's uterus was whole again, free of the masses that had stolen her peace for so long.

Jamie awoke groggy but safe. The catheter was unexpected and understandably alarming. I explained why it was needed, and she nodded slowly, processing everything.

"I didn't know it was that serious," she whispered. "But you saved it. You saved my uterus."

We removed the catheter during her two-week follow-up without complications or pain. Her healing had gone beautifully.

Jamie's body was finally free—no more bleeding, no more pain. She was no longer at the mercy of her fibroids. Today, she's healthy and thriving. She chose to have an IUD placed, not because she was trying to avoid pregnancy forever, but because she wanted to give her body time to rest and to protect that delicate reconnection we worked so hard to preserve.

She remains fibroid-free. And more than that, she remains full of hope.

More than a surgery

Jamie's story is a bold declaration: You are not wrong for wanting more for yourself.

If she had listened to that first opinion—or the second or third—she would have undergone a hysterectomy she didn't want.

Her uterus would be gone. Her choices would have been taken from her. And perhaps worst of all, she would have felt like her voice never mattered.

Instead, she kept fighting. She believed that her dreams were worth saving and they were.

Her journey is not just about fibroids. It's about advocacy. About trusting your gut when the world tells you to sit down and be quiet. It's about asking again, and again, and again until someone finally sees you—not just your diagnosis.

Jamie's story is proof that complex does not mean impossible. With the right care, even the most difficult cases can end in healing, wholeness, and renewed possibility.

And sometimes, that path starts with one brave woman refusing to accept "no" for an answer.

Precision and Preservation | 55

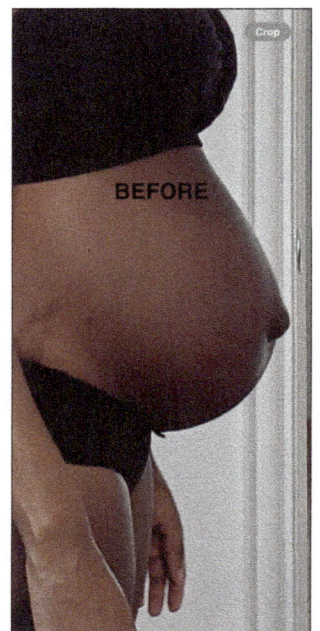

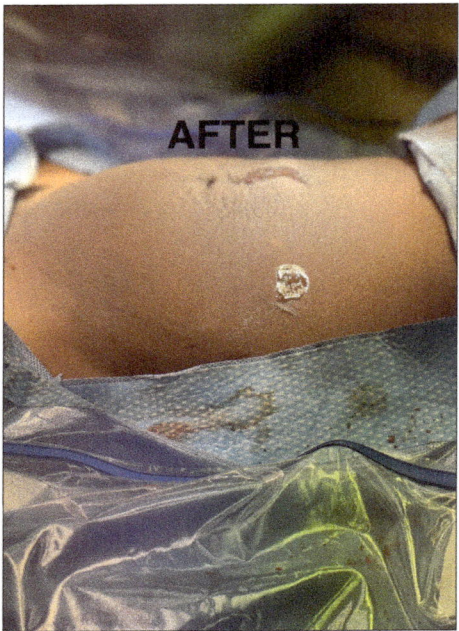

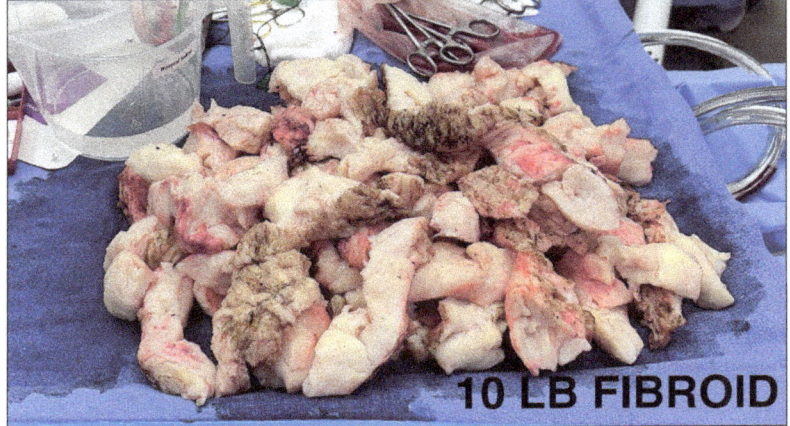

CHAPTER 10

The Silent Growth, and the Loud Dream

Not every woman with fibroids experiences debilitating pain, constant bleeding, or the unmistakable discomfort that so many others know all too well. For some, fibroids hide quietly in the background, unnoticed, unbothered, and undiagnosed. Jennifer Lee was one of those women.

In her early 40s, Jennifer was vibrant, driven, and ready to take on a new chapter in life—motherhood. She wasn't waiting for the "right time" or the "perfect partner." She was embarking on the journey of in vitro fertilization (IVF) using donor sperm.

Jennifer was full of hope and anticipation, imagining a life with lullabies, tiny socks, and first steps. But just as she was about to begin, her plans were halted by something invisible, silent, and surprisingly large: a 12-centimeter fibroid.

Jennifer had never experienced a single symptom, or so she thought. No painful periods. No heavy bleeding. No significant cramping.

Her body had never betrayed her before, and so when her fertility workup revealed a massive, pedunculated fibroid near the cervix, she was stunned. It was growing dangerously close to her right ureter, nestled in a region that could easily complicate pregnancy, let alone fertility treatment.

This wasn't supposed to be part of the story. She had never had surgery before. She had taken care of herself, trusted her body, and now she was being asked to press pause on the one thing she wanted most.

During our first consultation, Jennifer's guard was up—not in fear, but in determination. She had come too far to let this diagnosis derail her. Still, she questioned whether the fibroid was truly a problem. After all, she felt fine.

As we talked further, she slowly began to acknowledge symptoms she had brushed aside: mild urinary frequency, occasional pressure when sitting, subtle shifts in her body that she had chalked up to stress or aging. Looking back, she began to see the signs that had been hiding in plain sight.

Upon examining her, I confirmed what imaging had already shown—a large, mobile mass tucked deep in the posterior cul-de-sac, the hidden space behind the uterus and in front of the rectum. Though she had never noticed it, her body had been compensating for it all along.

I gently explained the risks of proceeding with IVF without addressing the fibroid—how its size and location could impair implantation, affect embryo growth, and even increase the risk of miscarriage.

Jennifer listened quietly, then took a breath and nodded. "Okay," she said. "Let's do the surgery. I want to give myself the best chance to become a mom."

Four months later, after completing her preoperative workup and preparing emotionally for her first-ever surgery, Jennifer entered the operating room. She was nervous, of course, but more than anything, she was hopeful. This wasn't just about fibroids. It was about fighting for her future.

Using the robotic surgical system, I began what I expected to be a fibroid removal. What I found was more than any scan had revealed.

In addition to the large pedunculated fibroid, Jennifer had endometriosis—implants scattered across her pelvis, clinging to her uterine walls and hiding behind her organs like tiny saboteurs. They had never been diagnosed, never caused pain, and yet there they were, possibly contributing to her fertility struggles in silence.

The surgery was anything but simple. The fibroid had grown from the lower uterine segment and right cervix, positioned perilously close to the uterine vessels and the ureter.

Every move required surgical finesse. But with the enhanced precision and visualization of the robotic platform, I was able to dissect around those critical structures without causing damage.

I removed two fibroids in total, the large one compressing the ureter and a smaller one embedded in the front of her uterus. Thankfully, neither required extensive uterine repair, which meant a quicker recovery and a safer path forward for fertility treatments.

Jennifer's resilience was remarkable. She was discharged that same day, and within a week, she was already easing back into her routine, defying the typical two-week recovery timeline. At her three-month follow-up, she was cleared for IVF. Her path to motherhood, once shadowed by doubt, was clear again.

Lessons from a quiet fighter

Jennifer's story is a powerful reminder that fibroids can be present without pain but still have a profound impact. It highlights why a comprehensive evaluation is so important, especially before starting fertility treatment.

For many women, IVF is an emotionally, physically, and financially taxing journey. To give themselves the best chance, the uterus must be in optimal condition. Jennifer's decision to address her fibroids before IVF was brave, proactive, and ultimately empowering.

Her story also reveals how minimally invasive, robotic-assisted surgery can transform outcomes. With precise movements and smaller incisions, we can navigate even the most complex pelvic anatomy, minimize trauma, and help women recover faster, so they can return to the things that matter most.

Reclaiming possibility, rewriting futures

The robotic platform has changed what is possible for women with fibroids. For many, it means the difference between a long hospital stay and a same-day discharge, between prolonged pain and a gentle recovery, and between delays in motherhood and moving forward with hope.

For Jennifer, surgery wasn't just about removing fibroids. It was about reclaiming her power, her body, and her dream. Her journey continues, IVF now back on track. And while the future is never guaranteed, she moves forward with the strength of knowing she did everything she could—boldly, courageously, and without regret.

And for every woman walking a similar path, Jennifer's story stands as a testament: Even in silence, even without symptoms, your body may be asking for help. Listen. Ask questions. Take action. Because motherhood, like healing, is rarely linear, but it is always worth fighting for.

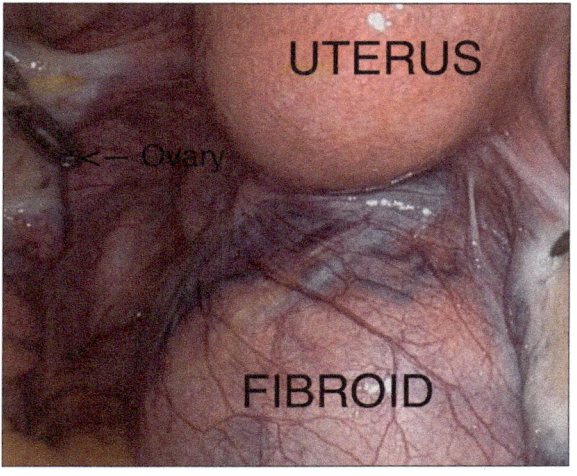

CONCLUSION

Breaking the Silence, Together

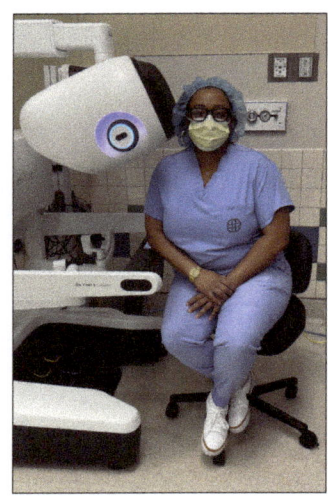

As we close this book, I want to speak to you directly, not as a surgeon or author, but as a witness to pain, a believer in healing, and a woman who has held the hands of countless others through their most vulnerable moments.

If you're here, you've walked with Ashley, Kellie, Felecia, Jamie, Sondra, Carla, Shante, and Jennifer. You've listened to their voices rise out of the silence, voices that have been muffled for too long by stigma, fear, and systemic neglect. You've seen the devastating effects of fibroids, but also the unimaginable strength of women who have taken back their power.

This book is more than information.

It's a movement. A mirror. A reckoning.

And it is only the beginning.

Throughout these chapters, you've learned about the debilitating symptoms of fibroids: the heavy bleeding, the crushing pelvic pressure, the fertility obstacles, the emotional toll. You've seen the difference that skilled, compassionate care can make. How minimally invasive surgeries, like robotic-assisted myomectomies and hysterectomies, can restore not just physical health, but a woman's sense of control and dignity.

We've also pulled back the curtain on the systemic issues that contribute to delayed diagnoses and subpar care, especially for women of color, who are more likely to have fibroids, to suffer more severe symptoms, and to be offered hysterectomy as a first resort.

We've challenged dangerous myths:

- That fibroids are "just part of being a woman."
- That pain is normal.
- That suffering is the price of femininity.

And we've shattered the silence by amplifying voices like:

Ashley, who endured years of misguided treatments and finally reclaimed her dream of becoming a mother with expert care.

Jamie, who held onto her desire of becoming a mother despite being told a hysterectomy was her only option.

Sondra, whose postmenopausal bleeding led to a rare but life-changing cancer diagnosis and who continues to fight with grace and grit.

Jennifer, who bravely prepared for IVF, only to uncover hidden challenges that required extraordinary precision and care.

Carla, who survived failed embolization, infection, and sepsis before finding healing through robotic surgery.

Kellie, who overcame shame and isolation, finding validation and hope in a surgical path tailored to her needs.

Shante, who fought to preserve her uterus and won when she was able to deliver 3 beautiful children, and then when she was ready, made the decision to take her life back by having a curative hysterectomy, proving that options, not ultimatums, should define care.

Felecia, who refused to settle for dismissive answers and kept searching until someone truly listened.

Each of these women is a chapter of truth, a testament to resilience, and a spark in a fire that is only growing.

You may be wondering, What now?

What do we do with all this truth?

The answer is simple but powerful: We act.

We cannot unknow what we've learned. We cannot turn away from the suffering that persists. So let's step forward, with purpose.

1. **Speak Up.**
   Start conversations. Share your story. Post about fibroids on social media. Host a book club. Send this book to your doctor. When we break the silence, we break the cycle of shame.

2. **Demand Better.**
   You deserve more than "wait and see." You deserve physicians who listen, options that are explained clearly, and access to advanced, minimally invasive care. Ask the hard questions. Get second and third opinions if necessary.

3. **Support the Mission.**
   Our fibroid foundation is committed to changing the narrative. We are building a future where:

   - Surgeries are accessible regardless of income or insurance.
   - Young girls are taught to recognize symptoms early.
   - An app connects women to accurate resources and vetted physicians.
   - No one feels invisible again.

4. **Hold Space for Others.**
   There is someone in your life right now who needs what you've just read. They may not have the words yet. They may not even know they're suffering from fibroids. Reach out. Ask questions. Listen. Be the hand they haven't found yet.

This book may end here, but our work is just beginning. If your heart has been moved, if you saw yourself or someone you love in these pages, I want to hear from you.

You are not just a reader. You are part of this story now. Part of this movement.

- **Email:** hopeandhealing@fibroidfreedom.org
- **Website:** www.fibroidfreedom.org
- **Social Media:** @drquanitacrable

We need your voice, your story, your passion. Together, we can create a future where fibroid care is no longer reactive but revolutionary.

To every woman who shared her story in these pages—thank you.

To every reader who chose to bear witness—thank you.

To everyone who is still suffering in silence—this book is for you.

I believe in a world where women are seen, believed, and healed. A world where suffering in silence is a thing of the past.

Let's build that world together.

With fierce hope and deep gratitude,
Dr. Quanita Crable
Surgeon. Advocate. Storykeeper.
Founder, **Hope and Healing: Fibroid Freedom Foundation**

Frequently Asked Questions (FAQ)

1. **What are fibroids, and how common are they?**
   Uterine fibroids are non-cancerous growths that develop from the muscle tissue of the uterus. They can vary in size, number, and location. Fibroids are incredibly common—up to 70-80% of women will develop them by age 50, though many may never know they have them. Black women are disproportionately affected, often developing fibroids earlier, with more severe symptoms and larger sizes.

2. **What causes fibroids?**
   The exact cause is unknown, but fibroids are influenced by hormones (especially estrogen and progesterone), genetics, and possibly environmental factors. Family history, early menstruation, obesity, and vitamin D deficiency may also increase risk. Stress and chronic inflammation are also being studied as contributing factors.

3. **What are the symptoms of fibroids?**
   Fibroid symptoms vary depending on size and location, but common symptoms include:

   - Heavy or prolonged menstrual bleeding
   - Pelvic pain or pressure
   - Frequent urination
   - Constipation or bloating
   - Pain during intercourse
   - Back or leg pain
   - Infertility or pregnancy complications

   Some women have no symptoms at all and discover fibroids incidentally during imaging.

4. **Can fibroids affect fertility or pregnancy?**
   Yes. Depending on their size and location, fibroids can interfere with conception, increase the risk of miscarriage, or lead to complications like preterm labor, breech presentation, or the need for cesarean delivery. Submucosal fibroids, those that grow into the uterine cavity, are most closely linked to fertility issues.

5. **Do fibroids always need to be removed?**
   No. Treatment depends on the severity of symptoms, size, and location of the fibroids, and whether a woman wants to preserve fertility. Asymptomatic fibroids often don't require treatment and can be managed with watchful waiting.

6. **What treatment options are available?**
   Treatment ranges from conservative to surgical:

   - Watchful waiting
   - Medications (e.g., birth control, GnRH agonists)
   - Minimally invasive procedures (UFE, MRgFUS, myomectomy)
   - Hysterectomy
   - Emerging treatments (radiofrequency ablation, SPRMs)

   See Chapter Two for a full breakdown of these options.

7. **Is hysterectomy the only permanent cure?**
   Yes, hysterectomy is the only treatment that completely eliminates the risk of fibroid recurrence. However, it's a major decision and not the only effective option. Many women successfully manage symptoms and preserve fertility with myomectomy or other treatments.

8. **Will my fibroids grow back after treatment?**
   If you don't have a hysterectomy, fibroids can potentially grow back or new ones can develop. This is more likely in women who are younger or have multiple fibroids. Myomectomy removes existing fibroids but does not prevent new ones from forming.

9. **Are fibroids cancerous?**
   The vast majority of fibroids are benign. In very rare cases (less than 1%), a cancerous tumor called leiomyosarcoma may be discovered. There's currently no reliable test to distinguish between benign and cancerous fibroids before surgery, which is why thorough evaluation and proper surgical techniques are critical.

10. **What questions should I ask my doctor?**
    Here are some key questions to consider:

    - What type of fibroids do I have, and where are they located?
    - How might the fibroids impact my fertility or pregnancy?
    - What are all of my treatment options?
    - What are the risks and benefits of each option?
    - What experience do you have with minimally invasive surgery?

    If you have any hesitations or unanswered questions, it is always a good idea to seek a second opinion.

11. **How do I find the right surgeon or fibroid specialist?**
    Seek a specialist who:

    - Listens to your concerns
    - Offers a range of treatment options (not just hysterectomy)
    - Has experience with minimally invasive or robotic surgery
    - Understands the impact of fibroids on fertility and quality of life

    It's okay to switch providers or get a second opinion until you feel fully supported.

12. **Can lifestyle changes help?**
    While lifestyle changes can't cure fibroids, they may help manage symptoms and reduce growth. These lifestyle updates can include:

    - Maintaining a healthy weight
    - Reducing consumption of red meat and increasing consumption of fruits, vegetables, and fiber
    - Getting adequate vitamin D
    - Adopting stress management techniques
    - Avoiding endocrine-disrupting chemicals when possible (e.g., in plastics, cosmetics)

13. **What emotional or mental health support is available?**
    Living with fibroids can be isolating, exhausting, and traumatic. You are not alone. Consider:

    - Support groups (in-person or online)
    - Mental health counseling
    - Patient advocacy groups
    - Books (like this one!) sharing stories and resources

    Your experience is valid and help is out there.

14. **What should I know if I'm nearing menopause?**
    Fibroids often shrink after menopause as hormone levels drop. If your symptoms are manageable, and you're close to menopause, a conservative approach may be appropriate. However, sudden bleeding or growth of a fibroid after menopause should always be evaluated, as it could signal something more serious.

15. **How can I support a loved one dealing with fibroids?**
    Offering support is one of the best things you can do.

    - Listen without judgment
    - Acknowledge their pain—emotional and physical
    - Help them navigate appointments, treatment decisions, or daily tasks
    - Advocate with them if they're not being heard
    - Share resources and encourage them to seek expert care

Resources

National Institutes of Health: https://pmc.ncbi.nlm.nih.gov/articles/PMC3136067/
U.S. Department of Health and Human Sources Office of Women's Health: https://womenshealth.gov/a-z-topics/uterine-fibroids
American College of Obstetricians and Gynecologists (ACOG): www.acog.com
World Health Organization (WHO): https://www.who.int/

About the Author

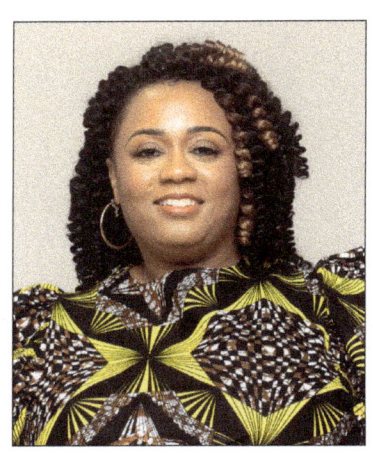

Dr. Quanita Crable is a board-certified OB/GYN specializing in minimally invasive gynecologic surgery, proudly serving women in the Dallas-Fort Worth area. With a focus on patient-centered care, she offers advanced treatment options for conditions such as abnormal menstrual bleeding, fibroids, ovarian cysts, pelvic pain, and pelvic organ prolapse. These options, including hysteroscopy, laparoscopy, and robotic-assisted surgery, allow for shorter hospital stays and faster recovery times.

Born in Pittsburgh, Pennsylvania and raised in Wichita, Kansas, Dr. Crable graduated from the University of Kansas with a degree in Chemistry. She went on to complete her medical degree at the University of Kansas School of Medicine and her residency in Obstetrics and Gynecology at KU Medical Center, where she received extensive training in minimally invasive techniques, including the da Vinci Surgical System.

Since relocating to Dallas in 2012, Dr. Crable has established her own practice dedicated to delivering exceptional patient care and providing patient education. She is deeply committed to building strong, respectful doctor-patient relationships and making every patient feel seen and heard.

Dr. Crable is a Junior Fellow of the American College of Obstetrics and Gynecology and a member of the American Association of Gynecologic Laparoscopists and the American Medical Association.

"It is a privilege to be trusted by women and their loved ones as they make decisions that impact their health. I have always been passionate about providing the quality of care that earns that trust."
– Dr. Quanita Crable

Reviews

"*Voices of Strength and Hope* is a powerful and deeply personal collection of stories from women navigating life with fibroids. Dr. Quanita Crable does something truly special—she listens. These are real stories from her patients, shared with honesty, pain, and ultimately, healing.

"What makes this book stand out is how Dr. Crable brings heart to healthcare. She doesn't just treat fibroids—she treats women.

"Alongside her patients' stories, Dr. Crable gently weaves in her own journey—from humble beginnings to becoming a leading OBGYN. Her path is one of determination and purpose, adding even more depth to the care she gives and the trust she builds.

"Reading this book felt like sitting with a group of brave women, hearing their struggles and triumphs. It's not just a medical book—it's a book on hope, resilience and the power of having a doctor who truly cares."

—***Tiffany S. Northern,*** *MHA, FACHE*
President of Texas Health Resources Frisco

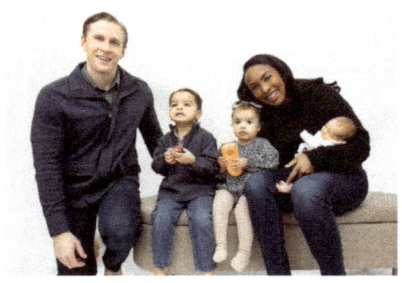

"I highly recommend this book to any woman who has given up on her dreams of having children because of fibroids. I've been there. I had two laparoscopic myomectomy surgeries—one to remove **33 fibroids,** another to remove 7—and thanks to the expertise and encouragement of Dr. Crable, my recovery was smooth and my hope was restored.

"Today, I'm the proud mother of **three healthy children,** all delivered safely by Dr. Crable via C-section. Her care gave me the confidence to believe in my body again, and this book will do the same for you."

—*Brit Rettig Wold*

"Dr. Crable beautifully captures the stories of real women from all seasons of life who, unfortunately, are familiar with the reality of fibroids.

"From Dr. Crable's journey to medicine to the courageous women who sought gynecological care from her, *Voices of Strength and Hope* is not only encouraging and hopeful but also informative. I stand in solidarity with these women, as I add my voice of hope and echo their sentiments. I too sought care from Dr. Crable and underwent minimally invasive robotic surgery to remove fibroids.

"I am so glad to have found a doctor who is not only an expert and specialist in gynecological care and surgery but also genuinely cares and has a passion for these specific ailments and concerns. My husband and I are so grateful to God for working through Dr. Crable, as I naturally conceived six months after undergoing

the procedure and welcomed a healthy baby boy without complication. Let this book reassure you that there are options and there is hope!"
—*Chloe*

"Dr. Crable is an excellent provider who has personally treated many of my patients who were suffering from both fibroids and infertility. She's an incredible and talented surgeon whom I feel proud to call both a respected colleague and a dear friend.
"From mission trips abroad to performing myomectomies in locations where access to basic health care is limited, to running her own practice and cultivating a safe space for her patients, Dr. Crable has always advocated for what's best for her patients.
"By sharing their stories, she is shedding light on a population's struggles that are often overlooked and forgotten. *Voices of Strength and Hope* is a culmination of the experience and wisdom she has gained over the years. I hope women suffering from fibroids can find comfort and knowledge in her words."
—*Dr. Tiffanny Jones*, M.D.
Reproductive Endocrinologist

"I just finished reading *Voices of Strength and Hope: Women's Stories of Overcoming Fibroids* by Dr. Quanita Crable, and I can confidently say it's a game-changer for anyone interested in women's health, particularly fibroids. This book, which is more like a memoir, isn't just informative; it's a heartfelt and beautifully written journey. Dr. Crable takes us on her personal journey to becoming a certified OB-GYN, the obstacles she overcame and the commitment she made to her grandmother. Her own story is one of strength, focus and determination and the dream of a 16-year-old girl who grew up to be the voice of others. Because of that commitment, we have a doctor rooted in Christ and using the gift He gave her to be a vessel to so many women.

"As someone always on the lookout for empowering stories and practical guidance, Dr. Crable's book completely blew me away. This book addresses the often-overlooked topic of fibroids with such grace and clarity.

"This book fills a crucial gap, offering not just information, but the personal touch that so many women are not afforded because we go unheard and unseen. What truly sets this book apart is Dr. Crable's commitment to empowering women to advocate for their own health, providing them with the knowledge to make informed decisions.

"I highly recommend this book to any woman who has been diagnosed with fibroids, suspects she might have them, or to anyone who simply wants to be more informed about women's reproductive health. It's also a valuable resource for partners, family members, and healthcare providers.

"Do yourself a favor and pick up a copy of *Voices of Strength and Hope*. It's more than just a book, but more of a much-needed guide on compassionate, patient-centered care that we don't always find."

—**LaDawna Crittenton McKinney,** *MHA, BSN, RNC-IAP.*
Best-selling Author
Clinical Nurse Supervisor, Antepartum Specialty Unit

"In my career as a physician who has the honor of taking care of infants admitted to the neonatal intensive care unit, a major perk of my job includes getting to know the background of the parents of my strong and resilient patients. I have heard countless stories from several families, as well as my own friends and family members, on the impact fibroids have had on their physical and mental health, especially when it has impacted their dreams of being parents.

"In *Voices of Strength and Hope,* Dr. Crable has seamlessly provided a voice for the often-dismissed faction of women who are often suffering in silence. Readers will delight in getting to know each character as they triumph against all odds. I am optimistic that this book will continue to open doors to aid in diagnosis for some and provide hope for a healthier future for all."

—Maya Heath, *M.D.*
Neonatologist

www.ingramcontent.com/pod-product-compliance
Lightning Source LLC
Chambersburg PA
CBHW052033030426
42337CB00027B/4991